FOCUS ON YOURSELF

FOCUS ON YOURSELF

A Holistic Healing Guide for
Inner Healing and Self-Discovery

Tiarra Abu-Bakr

ISBN: 979-8-218-14822-5

Because of the dynamic nature of the internet, any web addresses or links contained in this book may have changed since publication and may no longer be valid. The views expressed in this book are solely those of the author and do not necessarily reflect the views of the publisher, and the publisher disclaims any responsibility for them.

Printed it in the United States of America.

DEDICATIONS

This book is dedicated to the Goddess who gave me life, Robin Hayes. You are the reason I am. Your unwavering determination, resilient heart, and earthly wisdom provided me with the road map to discover myself. You endured so that I may soar, and there are not enough words to express my gratitude. I want to give you your flowers now: Thank you, Mom.

To my king, Jeremiah Abu Bakr, and our little ones; I appreciate your patience while I have been navigating this journey of self-discovery. My heart's purpose is to make your lives better. You all are what motivates me to keep working toward wellbeing. I am incredibly appreciative that I get to share my world with you.

TABLE OF CONTENTS

INTRODUCTION

I'm grateful that you are allowing me to share in your quest for self-discovery. The fact that you are holding this book in your hands means the world to me. It represents your awareness and motivation to transform your life. I don't know whether you know this, but awareness is the first step in the process of change. Before we embark on this journey, I would love the opportunity to allay any concerns. The terms "holistic healing" and "holistic wellbeing," will be used interchangeably in this text. I know sometimes the term "holistic" comes with some stigma around it, which is why I am excited about providing education and clarity around the subject.

Do you mind if I'm open with you? The publication of this book was attempted to be sabotaged by a variety of thoughts, feelings, and emotions as well as roadblocks and old thought patterns. I must let you know that I am my first client. Patient 0 is me. I'm still putting a lot of effort into figuring out all the different aspects of who I am. The fact that I'm writing this book doesn't indicate that I've succeeded, what it does indicate is that I've established a routine for learning about myself. Also, I have a reliable toolkit that I use when I find myself in tight spaces. Sharing my toolkit with you is an honor.

My journey of self-discovery and introduction to holistic healing began at the age of 24, following a broken marriage. In retrospect, I shouldn't have been married because I didn't know anything about myself. I was a people-pleaser with emotional processing issues. I couldn't even open my mouth to conduct a civilized, emotional discourse because the words became stuck in my throat. There was no way for me to advocate for myself or articulate my demands because I was unaware of them. That was a complete train wreck, and I'm glad I can look back and take responsibility for my mess.

If you're anything like I used to be, you've picked up this book because you're exhausted. You're sick of just existing. You have followed all of society's advice, but the results are not what you had anticipated. You come through for folks. You are trustworthy and accountable. You are goal-oriented and competent. Yet you still feel invisible, empty, and defeated. Most likely, you feel undervalued and cut off from the outside world. These emotions are so familiar to me because they were formerly my closest companions. They are the consequences of routinely engaging in self-neglect. Self-neglect and people-pleasing behaviors are not naturally occurring habits. I can guarantee that the conduct is related to a specific childhood experience.

I've worked as a direct service provider in more than ten different settings for almost 20 years. Many of my clients have experienced a recurrent problem: being sent out into the world without the time or chance to safely investigate themselves. As our personalities have changed because of stress and trauma, many people don't know who they are. We are unsure of how to interact with people most effectively or what we would do in life if there were no obstacles. In essence, we are unsure of who we are. You can use this book to help set the groundwork for your journey to discover yourself. And when I say journey, I really mean it; as you peel back the layers of your existence, you'll keep evolving, and eventually, you'll get to know your true self.

Are you prepared to meet the most authentic version of yourself? If so, I want to give you some advice. Don't rush the process. I rarely look back on my life with regret. Yet, I'm willing to admit that every time I hurried through a process, I significantly missed something. For instance, I rushed through the process when I was a graduate student. I wanted it to be over quickly so I could get to my life as a therapist. However, there is a purpose to why they put you in a cohort. That voyage should not be undertaken by one person. The closest people to me were unable to truly support or understand my challenges since they had never been in my shoes. Because I had not connected with my designated cohort by the time that season in my life ended, I was worn out and failed to pass my clinical examinations. I was in a rush and missed some critical elements of the journey. Obviously, I eventually passed, hence my current role as a therapist. My advice is to allow yourself full access to the experience. As you peel back the layers of who you are, take your time with the thoughts, feelings, and realizations you encounter. And sit in it for some time; don't stay there, but experience it.

Be aware that everyone's experience of healing is unique. Take what strikes a chord with you and discard the items that don't. This is not a scenario where one solution fits all. Some of the tactics in this book used to work like magic for me, but they no longer do. You could have a similar experience. Without passing judgment, move through it and keep learning what works for you. The only failure is not giving yourself the chance to know yourself; you cannot fail at discovering yourself. You deserve this season of YOU. The life of your dreams is within your grasp. You can create that life. What would that life entail?

Finally, let's discuss what you can expect in this book: You will receive parts of my journey that address sexual assault, homelessness, domestic violence, and suicidal ideation (trigger warning). Additionally, there are exercises in the book that will request you to explore your traumatic experiences. Please honor yourself by taking breaks as needed. Each chapter provides you with one of my favorite inspirational quotes, insight on the pillars of wellness, a lesson to implement, a strategy to add to your toolkit, and moment of reflection to assist you with processing what was digested. You will need: an open mind, a mirror, a dry erase marker (or sticky notes), and honesty. If you do the work, this journey can be life altering. You should expect to unveil some things about yourself that were hidden. I suggest working with a mental health therapist if you experience overwhelming emotional stress.

MOMENT OF REFLECTION
WHO ARE YOU?

Task 1

Get out a dry erase marker. Please take a seat in front of a mirror (a full length one is preferred but not essential) so you can see yourself. If your hair, scars, or extra weight are upsetting you, look pass them in this moment. Let go of your judgment and concentrate on penning your observations, using the mirror as your canvas.

It's crucial to evaluate your condition at the beginning of your journey to properly accept your evolution.

Who are you at this moment?

_____
_____
_____
_____

How do you feel about the person you just observed in the mirror?

_____
_____
_____
_____

Describe the qualities of the woman you desire to become.

_____

_____

_____

_____

CHAPTER 1
THE RESIDUE OF TRAUMA

"Childhood trauma can lead to an adulthood spent in survival mode, afraid to plant roots, to plan for the future, to trust, and to let joy in. It's a blessing to shift from surviving to thriving. It's not simple but there is more than survival."

— Unknown

Growing up, moving was a very common occurrence in my life. I'm unable to count the moves with any degree of accuracy, but I can clearly remember one of the most unforgettable moments. At the time, we were staying with my mother's boyfriend's sister. Her home was tidy, warm, and welcoming. Up until that point, it seemed stable. I can recall being startled awake in the middle of the night. "Hurry and get dressed, pack your clothes in a trash bag, and let's go," my mother said. I understood this was not the appropriate time to inquire about what was happening. I knew I should just do what I was told. Nevertheless, my 7-year-old brain could already comprehend what was going on. We had to leave since my mother and her boyfriend had a major argument. We boarded a cab, put everything we owned into garbage bags, and arrived at an office building.

We were in an after-hours social service facility. My siblings and I received blankets so we could rest on the floor while they assisted my mother with the intake procedure. The procedure seemed to take an eternity. They were asking her things like, "What other resources do you have available?" "Is there a different relative you can stay with?" Everywhere, the response was the same: "No." We lacked both resources and assistance. We were put in a shelter after a lengthy admission process. The unforgettable portion comes next. This location was a room designed to accommodate a family of six. There were, however, only two beds. We were accustomed to sleeping in tight quarters, so it wasn't a huge concern.

We got in bed to sleep for a few hours because everyone was completely worn out and we had to leave the shelter as the sun rose. I heard mice and rats scratching the walls as I was about to close my eyes and drift off. I was in bed with my mother and sister closest to the wall. To say that I was terrified is an understatement. I chose to spend hours standing in the middle of the floor while the sun rose because I wouldn't sleep on that bed. Even though standing in the center of the floor was equally awful, there was no way I was going to let those rats approach me before I could stomp them out. Although this story is now amusing, it had a profound impact on my life. As soon as it was time to depart, we rummaged through the bags of clothing, changed into our clothes, and arrived at school as if nothing had happened the previous night. To us, it was normal. I can think of several instances where the chemistry of my brain cells was altered. Trauma leaves a legacy that lingers for generations.

Frequent moves as a child are linked to low adult quality of life, especially in introverted people, according to an article published in the June issue of the Journal of Personality and Social Psychology. According to the study, people who moved frequently as adults had fewer healthy connections. The more moves an introvert makes, the worse off they are as adults. The study reports that individuals who moved around often in childhood were more likely to pass away sooner than the other study participants. There is concern that moving causes stress, and stress has a bad impact on people's health, even though the relationship between frequent relocation and lifespan cannot be proven.

The word trauma tends to create some confusion. People often think of trauma as an event or experience. Trauma is the emotional reaction to a traumatic or life-changing occurrence that leaves a person with long-lasting impacts on their physical, mental, emotional, and spiritual health. Extroverts, for instance, are said to be less likely to be negatively affected by numerous moves as a child since they are more able to form friendships and positive connections. For me, relocating often and being introverted created a social and emotional sense of unsafety and instability that still shows up in adulthood. This is the residue of my trauma, and it requires me to intentionally do the work of maintaining relationships. When my mind tells me to retreat because it is unsafe, I must intentionally practice holding onto relationships.

I still have a terrible fear of rats and mice because of what I saw during that time of moving. My body has a visceral reaction when I see or hear them. I immediately feel queasy, and I'll never forget that night in the shelter. I have, however, developed a strong self-care strategy that enables me to ground myself when my body begins to recall traumatic experiences. Even though my kids were never in the shelter with me, I could easily pass along this similar phobia of rodents to them. Yet, by learning to calm myself, I can safely work through my trauma reactions and prevent others from having the same fear-based reactions I did. This is the aftermath of trauma. We adopt a coping strategy after observing it in our parents, families, and communities. We go through life replicating the behaviors that were modeled for us unless someone intervenes and points out the anomalies or risks in our lifestyles.

I'm not a huge fan of science. Nevertheless, finding out about the ground-breaking ACES study, which was conducted at Kaiser Permanente in 1995, changed my life. Adverse Childhood Experiences Study (ACES) looked at the connection between self-reported childhood trauma and adult health. The types of trauma examined in this study were parental separation, parental mental illness, parental substance misuse, parental incarceration, child abuse, child neglect, and general household dysfunction. The study's two key conclusions were that adverse childhood experiences are widespread, even among middle class groups. Most people go through some kind of traumatic experience as a child; some people go through three or more traumatic experiences. Second, there was a direct link between childhood trauma and negative adult outcomes like heart disease, diabetes, obesity, depression, subpar academic performance, smoking, and even premature mortality.

I was startled when I finished the examination of myself. There are 10 questions in the evaluation, and each yes receives one point. I received an ACES score of nine. This suggests that I have a high likelihood of acquiring heart disease or another chronic illness, becoming a victim of domestic abuse, developing a mental health condition, and passing away at a young age. Just like many of us, I made it through everything I went through as a child. But we cannot confuse survival for wellness. This study demonstrates that the effects of trauma are much more severe than some of the early encounters we may have.

I entered the field of holistic wellness because of this study. While the ACES study is accurate, it does not constitute a death warrant. I have the chance to cure myself and work toward optimum wellness every day that I take a breath. I urge you to assess your ACES score and sort through the traumatizing remnants. Find the facets of your personality that grew because of something painful. Find the aspects of yourself that are still concealed because they couldn't safely emerge. Make a list of how you are currently treating your body. Do you suffer from any illnesses that may be linked to the trauma your family has suffered in the past? It's likely that your way of living is taking even more years off you. The strategy for reclaiming your years and efficiently controlling your quality of life while you're still here is holistic wellness.

I'm ecstatic to provide you with a thorough explanation of holistic wellbeing. I hope you use this book as a tool in your quest for healing. Remember that not everything expressed in this space may be appropriate for you, as I have stated. Although it may not be a part of your practice, being knowledgeable of various healing modalities is advantageous since you will have the knowledge to impart to someone else who may be looking for ways to heal themselves. This is how the community regains its power. Join me in the following chapter as we explore holistic wellness in more detail.

Lesson: Don't just be aware of the traumatic experiences you have survived. Become a student of yourself and discover how those experiences shaped you.

For Your Toolkit: Holistic Therapy

For a variety of mental and emotional issues, holistic therapy uses methods that are non-traditional of mainstream, conventional care. Like other types of psychotherapy, holistic psychotherapy is effective. It adopts a whole-person approach that stresses treating and enhancing all facets of a person's life rather than focusing on just one area of their health. An integrated approach combines traditional and complementary therapies, such as psychotherapy, medicine, acupuncture, and yoga.

We talk about life events, stressors, memories, thought patterns, and other things that are influencing our clients' mental health during treatment. However, unlike more conventional forms of psychotherapy, holistic psychotherapy also addresses issues related to the body and the spirit. When our minds are suffering, so do our bodies and spirits. We may create plans to heal each of these components by identifying the ways that our mental health affects our bodies and souls. We lose out on significant healing opportunities that result in more substantial and long-lasting transformation if we simply target the mind.

MOMENT OF REFLECTION
YOUR RESIDUE

Task 2

Spend some time exploring the most traumatic experiences you have survived and the triggers that linger as a result.

_____

_____

_____

_____

To pull up the root, delve below the surface.

_____

_____

_____

_____

Share how these traumatic events changed your personality and sense of self.

_____

_____

_____

_____

CHAPTER 2
WHAT IS HOLISTIC WELLNESS?

"Health is a state of complete harmony of the body, mind, and spirit. When one is free from physical disabilities and mental distractions, the gates of the soul open."

– B.K.S. Iyengar

The approach to wellness known as holistic healing encompasses all facets of wellbeing. It is a type of healing that considers the entire individual. The nine pillars of wellness—emotional, social, environmental, spiritual, financial, intellectual, physical, creative, and sexual wellness—are utilized throughout this work. Later in the book, we shall discuss each of these pillars separately. It's incredible that healing is in style today, but I believe it's crucial to recognize the interconnectivity of each of the pillars. I have seen many clients actively working to improve their mental health while attempting to preserve problematic social networks in the mistaken belief that this will allow them to maintain optimum wellness. Unhealthy social environments do, in fact, eventually permeate your state of being. A disease that resides in any of the pillars must be treated similarly because it will inevitably spread.

I'm not suggesting that the resolution is to disconnect from everyone and everything. I'm telling you to evaluate every aspect of your life. Determine the disease's origin and try to develop systems that help you live healthily. Various resources can be used in conjunction with holistic wellness. When researching your own body and combining the proper foods, herbs, and supplements that provide you optimal health, you can and should engage the help of a medical expert. You can engage in breath work to let go of stored energy while praising God from dawn to dusk. This way of life emphasizes 'yes…and' rather than 'either…or.' This is about accepting personal responsibility to raise your standard of living, and you get to decide how.

Many modalities outside of holistic wellness work in compartments, yet that is not how our bodies function. When you are worried about the state of your finances, stress does not identify it as just a financial problem and isolate concern to your bank account. Your body harbors that financial stress, which ultimately impacts your quality of life. Developing habits that enable you to properly identify, address, release, and mend are key to holistic wellness. In this lifetime, everything we go through is a mind, body, spirit, and soul interaction. So that we can stop engaging in self-neglect, it is essential that we navigate this life holistically. You are engaging in self-neglect if you don't regularly assess yourself using the nine pillars as you go through life.

Since holistic living is so much more than just a method for healing trauma, it would be unjust of me to reduce it to that. The process of self-discovery is what makes holistic wellness and healing so beautiful. Let's face it, many of us are exactly who our parents told us to be. I stated in the introduction that I had experience working as a therapist in many contexts. And I'll say it again: most of the people I've helped had the same background. They were a mystery to them. I believe that sentiment is one that we have all experienced at some point in our lives, and for some of us, it is still present today. Setting up your framework for how you want to conduct your life using the nine pillars is a productive idea because self-discovery can seem unattainable, especially if you don't have a framework to work within.

The most common sentence I hear from clients in my work with them—and the inspiration for this book—is "I don't know who I am, and I don't know how to find out." To experience wellbeing in all spheres, my goal was to establish a space where people could go deep into uncovering their trauma, working through it, and then getting to the essence of who they are. I'm overjoyed for you if you're reading this and getting motivated about coordinating your life with this holistic path. As this book offers you guidance, I don't want you to stress or worry about how it will turn out or how you will go about doing it. More importantly, I want you to understand that this is a journey and that it won't finish until you have fulfilled your mission in this world. Let's start by learning more about the nine pillars of wellness.

Lesson: Realize that you are a complex person with many layers. You have an obligation to be aware of the state of your health. That requires continual assessment of your entire being.

For Your Toolkit: Chakra Balancing

Our centers of consciousness are known as chakras. They store the vitality of our ideas, feelings, encounters, and memories. Your experiences are created by the energy that is stored in your chakras. Chakra balance can help you feel better because your body is a physical representation of your spirit. It is possible for a chakra to be balanced, underactive, or overactive. Depending on our experiences, perspectives, and physical health, it may be flowing at a healthy pace, sluggish, or blocked. A chakra can become blocked for a variety of reasons, but the most typical one is an unhealthy lifestyle. A blocked chakra is primarily caused by excessive stress, bad thinking, a lack of exercise, insufficient sleep, and an improper diet.

The technique of chakra balancing involves removing obstructions and restoring a healthy rate of chakra flow. How you feel and interact with the conditions in your life depends on the condition of your chakras and energy field. With the help of chakra balancing, we may take care of our consciousness and discover the lessons we are meant to learn before they show up as disease or loss. Chakras that are in balance promote both mental and emotional health.

Each of the seven primary chakras corresponds to a certain body part, including organs and glands. They interact with the neurological and endocrine systems after passing through the physical body. In an energy healing session, you might feel or visualize the spinning wheels even though you can't see them in the physical form.

- At the base of your spine is the first chakra, often known as the Root Chakra. Red is the color that it belongs to.
- The sacral chakra, the second chakra, is found in the region of the pelvis. Orange is the hue that goes with it.
- The Solar Plexus Chakra, the third chakra, is situated in the middle of your abdomen. Yellow is the color that it goes with.
- Your heart, or the fourth chakra, is situated in the middle of your chest. It relates to green.
- The center of your throat is where the Throat Chakra, the fifth chakra, is situated. It relates to blue.
- Your forehead's center holds the Third Eye Chakra, which is the sixth chakra. Indigo is the hue that goes with it.
- The crown, or Crown Chakra, is home to your seventh chakra. Its corresponding hues are violet and white.

MOMENT OF REFLECTION
RATE YOUR WELLNESS

Task 3

Use the scale to take inventory of your wellness within the nine pillars. Then briefly explain what you believe needs to happen for you to improve the current rating. You should aim to get to rating five (5) overtime. However, note that this takes time and work. If you can move from rating one(1) to two(2) then three(3), you are making progress. Honor that progress.

5 - Optimal Wellness: I am excelling in this area.
4 - Generally Well: I am not perfect in this area, but I am consistent.
3 – Maintaining: I am doing some things well, but I can do better.
2 - Barely Making It: I am trying but I'm struggling.
1 - Absolute Distress: I am not holding space for this area of my life at all.

Emotional Wellness:

_____

_____

_____

_____

Social Wellness:

_____

_____

_____

_____

Environmental Wellness:

_____

_____

_____

_____

Spiritual Wellness:

_____

_____

_____

_____

Financial Wellness:

_____

_____

_____

_____

Intellectual Wellness:

_____
_____
_____
_____

Physical Wellness:

_____
_____
_____
_____

Creative Wellness:

_____
_____
_____
_____

Sexual Wellness:

_____
_____
_____
_____

CHAPTER 3
EMOTIONAL WELLNESS

"The cheerful mind perseveres, and the strong mind hews its way through a thousand difficulties."
— Swami Vivekananda

The years between third and sixth grade were the most stable for me when I was younger. We spent a significant amount of time living in one place throughout this period. I had established a solid network of close friends, along with solid ties to the faculty and administration in my school. In fact, one of my teachers would routinely replenish any lacking supplies. She never questioned me; all she did was offer food or clothing for me to take home. She genuinely cared for me. We relocated during the middle of the sixth-grade year to a location that seemed extremely far away at the time—keeping in mind that cell phones weren't common at that time. So, bidding farewell felt like goodbye forever. We've already talked about how tough it is for introverts to stay in relationships.

I, therefore, feared that there was no way I could keep up those friendships and connections with the distance.

My mother moved the family into a gorgeous new house. I remember being in my bedroom alongside my older sisters as we were unpacking and setting up our space. I was grateful to my mother for taking us out of dangerous conditions and placing us in a stable area. But I recall feeling so torn and so sad inside because my sense of stability was gone. As we were unpacking, a song came on the radio that sent me spiraling. I still remember the lyrics: "Count on me through thick and thin, a friendship that will never end, when you are weak, I will be strong, helping you to carry on, call on me I will be there. Don't be afraid, please believe me when I say count on me." The words in the song cut through my 11-year-old body so deeply that I immediately started crying uncontrollably.

I was indeed the target of my sisters' loud laughter as they observed my emotional display. They were acting like teenagers at the time, as we were all rather young. But that experience was so impactful for me. I made a pledge to myself at that time to never again show that level of vulnerability to anyone. And I clung tenaciously to that promise. I didn't cry again for another ten years. I restrained myself from crying. I was unable to cry, even when I needed to. I recall the agony of going through a divorce as my small family broke apart; as hurt as I was, I couldn't bring myself to cry. I didn't start accessing my emotions again until I purposefully focused on my own healing and gave myself permission to reclaim that element of myself. Refusing to be vulnerable felt like a good strategy for self-protection. It was the biggest contributor to my self-neglect. And it created a huge sense of disconnection from myself and the world around me. And for a portion of my adult life, my emotional maturity and intelligence were on par with the 11-year-old kid who was emotionally wounded.

The capacity to be aware, understanding, and accepting of one's feelings is referred to as emotional wellbeing. It is the capacity to successfully navigate and control changes and problems in life. Our lives are significantly impacted by our emotional well-being. A person is more likely to have trouble handling other people's emotions if they lack the abilities necessary to effectively regulate their own emotions. In addition to harming our interpersonal connections, emotional instability also has a cascading effect on our mental health. Ignoring emotions can result in memory problems, a weakened immune system, high blood pressure, more mental difficulties, and low productivity, which can affect performance at work and in the classroom. Most crucially, a person's capacity to bounce back from setbacks in life is impacted by their emotional equilibrium.

Laying a strong foundation for your ideal home is analogous to improving your mental wellness. By making emotionally healthy decisions rather than relying on trauma-based reactions, you can succeed in life by maintaining consistent emotional wellness. Those who are emotionally stable are conscious of their stress levels and have a good technique for taking care of their emotions. I have a few suggestions for you if you're attempting to figure out how to improve your emotional wellness. First, evaluate your life. Where does the tension originate? Is the cause of your stress essential to your existence? What keeps you from releasing it if anything? If it is essential, create a plan for how you want to deal with the stressor.

Second, give yourself permission to set appropriate boundaries. Are you overworking your relationships and yourself? Do you balance your work and personal life well? Are you in good friendships? Do you regularly employ a no-boundaries policy in situations where emotional imbalance is present? Finally, be vulnerable and cultivate mindfulness. Likewise, be honest with yourself. With other people, being honest is desirable, but lying to yourself makes it impossible to be honest with others. Any feelings that arise, be completely honest with yourself about them, even when it feels repulsive. Remember that emotional wellness is the foundation for your wellness, and you want to build on solid ground.

Lesson: Identify, name, and process the feeling. You cannot continue to practice avoidance of your feelings. Furthermore, avoidance doesn't make it disappear. It gives it permission to linger.

For Your Toolbox: Transparent Journaling

Journaling in a way that demands you to be brutally honest with yourself is known as transparent journaling. When we're worried about someone reading or finding out what's truly going on inside of us, we withhold information, write only partially, or reveal only a portion of what's coming up for us. As a result, we are left with residual feelings that are unresolved and whose potential we haven't properly explored. You allow yourself to thoroughly explore all the concepts that are coming up for you as you write as though no one will ever read what you're writing. It greatly aids because, once you fully permit yourself to analyze the thought, it dissipates rather than remaining inside of your head where it might fester, develop, and bring shame.

MOMENT OF REFLECTION
EMOTIONAL AVOIDANCE

Task 4

There are some emotions that can feel so intense that we tend to avoid them. Unfortunately, avoiding emotions can keep them at high intensity. The most intense feelings are listed below, take some time to identify how you currently process these emotions. Take some time to write out your responses below.

Hate:

Anger:

Sadness:

Jealousy:

Resentment:

Fear:

Loneliness:

Longing:

Now that you have processed the way you move through these difficult emotions, which emotion would you like to see yourself managing differently?

_____

_____

_____

_____

CHAPTER 4
SOCIAL WELLNESS

"The meeting of two personalities is like the contact of two chemical substances: if there is any reaction, both are transformed."

– Carl Jung

I've been able to analyze and recognize that I frequently felt out of place as a child and that social interaction was overwhelming most of the time. I felt strangely different and as if I didn't fit in any of the settings. Throughout middle school, I learned how to disguise my emotions of exclusion by changing my personality to blend in. I was able to fit into the clique of popular girls, also known as the mean girls. I joined in on the everyday name-calling and derogatory remarks that we made at other girls because I was so happy to have found a tribe. I didn't communicate with that group of girls after middle school because those connections weren't rooted in substance.

The full circle moments that life presents to us are often entertaining. Years later, I was sitting at my administrative assistant position getting ready for the daily flow of interviews the company would perform. One of the candidates, who I remembered from middle school, arrived, and greeted me. I was so eager to see her that I even remembered her name. I greeted her enthusiastically and asked how her life had been going. She didn't seem to want to talk to me, which was obvious. I contributed her distance to anxiety about the interview, and I went back to my desk to give her time to collect her thoughts.

After finishing her interview, she came to my desk to explain how I had treated her in middle school in such a horribly unpleasant way. I was one of her bullies in her eyes, she said. I suddenly understood that I would have done anything to fit in with that group of girls because I wanted to be a part of them so badly. I ruined another person's emotional state. I apologized. And I made the decision to assess my social wellbeing at that point. This experience was a true reflection of how childhood trauma lingers into adulthood because it did for both of us. Realizing that I was a bully unearthed some things about my thought process regarding friendship. I developed a deep sense of mistrust for other women because of it. My conviction was that if we sat around and denigrated people, the same thing would happen when I stepped away from the group. My position in that group of girls contributed to my growing sense of insecurity. Even though I yearned to fit in, being alone felt safer.

Without addressing the significance of social wellness, it is impossible to take a complete approach to your health and wellbeing.

Let's describe social wellness in detail. The ability to build and maintain relationships with people and to communicate effectively within those interactions is referred to as social wellbeing. By cultivating meaningful connections, you can feel genuine, appreciated, connected, and like you belong. Because they enable you to feel noticed and valued, these interactions have a big impact. Our urge to be with people is caused by the limbic system in the brain. We depend on one another because we are social beings.

Your social support system should make you feel secure and at ease, not uneasy. This is the moment to evaluate your role in any unhealthy or exhausting relationships you may be in. Gossiping, judging people, and being critical of others are all self-destructive behaviors. It's crucial to be in accepting, constructive, and nurturing relationships to sustain a good level of social wellbeing. These are some strategies for developing wholesome social connections: Devote time to the relationship. Be open and encouraging of one another's emotions, aspirations, and dreams. Refrain from blaming and criticizing each other for communication errors. Stop trying to fix people. Show your appreciation in both spoken and nonverbal ways. Use clarifying language instead of hasty judgment. In your relationships, strike a balance between giving and taking. Instead of competing, celebrate.

While our social networks can change as we get older, certain intimate ties stay and grow with us. Friendships and relationships may ebb and flow as we mature in self-awareness and authenticity. This is a typical feature of life, even though it can be difficult to understand. Make sure to develop the habit of checking in with yourself when your relationships change. To fill the void with reality rather than supposition, process your feelings with the other person. Working for connections that you value is acceptable, and letting go of relationships that feel harmful to your wellbeing is also acceptable. I advise you to think about yourself and how you have contributed to the state of the relationship before you start blaming the other person.

Lesson: The quality of your tribe matters because your relationships serve as a mirror for you. If your relationships feel out of alignment, explore yourself to find out why.

For Your Toolbox: Reiki Healing

Reiki is a Japanese term that translates as "universal lifeforce energy." It's a method of holistically treating your mind, body, and spirit. Reiki works to balance and unblock the body's energy centers and promote healing. As a result, the energy is directed to the areas of the body, mind, emotions, and spirit that need it. Reiki treats any disease's root cause, not just its symptoms. Many people notice an improvement after only one Reiki treatment. During the session, a Reiki practitioner rests their hands slightly above your body in the regions of your chakras to help you feel peaceful and relaxed. Sessions may last anywhere between 20 and 90 minutes. Deep relaxation is achieved by Reiki. It aids in easing pain and stress, accelerating the healing of wounds, and enhancing your general health.

People use Reiki to treat stress and anxiety, depression, post-traumatic stress disorder (PTSD), low mood, trouble sleeping, and relationship difficulties because it supports and celebrates the body's innate ability to heal itself while reducing pain, removing toxins, and creating balance throughout one's entire energy field. Reiki also challenges you to reflect on your emotional reactions and let go of unfavorable feelings like resentment and wrath. If you're attempting to become more deliberate about cultivating more social consciousness and wellness in your life, this is a lovely practice to include. Reiki can aid in self-awareness and the development of more useful reactions, both of which will enhance the quality of your relationships in general.

IDENTIFYING SOCIAL THEMES

Task 5

Now is the time to identify the social themes in your life. Reflect on your childhood, what was the messaging around relationships and friendships?

_____

_____

_____

_____

How important are social connections to you?

_____

_____

_____

_____

Are your current relationships/friendships healthy? Are there con-versations that you are avoiding?

_____

_____

_____

_____

What recurring challenges have you experienced in your social connections?

_____

_____

_____

_____

CHAPTER 5
ENVIRONMENTAL WELLNESS

"The major problems in the world are the result of the difference between how nature works, and the way people think."

— Gregory Bateson

Environmental wellbeing entails valuing the connection between ourselves, the environments in which we reside and work, and the world. The fundamental tenet of environmental wellbeing is respect for all of nature and the creatures that inhabit it. You will be able to understand how your daily behaviors affect your life at home and at work once you become environmentally conscious. Environmental wellness includes taking care of your home and business premises. As a result, you become more productive and stress-free.

As I worked in the DC correctional facility, environmental wellness was introduced into my consciousness. DC Jail is a facility that houses a very low and sad frequency, in terms of energy. There is a strong sense of lifelessness caused by the dim lighting, terrible smells, loud noises, guards, and prison bars. I genuinely enjoyed working with the citizens (offenders). I had a terrific working relationship with the male returning citizens population. But I started to notice how much of an impact the environment was having on my physical health after I had been working in the facility for almost two years. And I essentially had to hold my breath every day as I was going into work. There was no access to the outside world and a constant sense of hyper-awareness would jump on me when the facility's doors slammed closed. Every time I clocked out of work, a huge sigh of relief escaped my body. Fortunately, I was permitted to leave the institution each day and go back to my house. Nonetheless, the detainees were required to occupy this space under the fictitious guise of recovery and rehabilitation.

Environmental wellness plays a significant role in your wellbeing and that encompasses the state of your house, the level of clutter, air quality, and chemical use. Also, it is important to remember that the conditions of your working environment are directly correlated to your mental health. I recognize that we are not always granted the privilege to be picky about our employment opportunities. If that is the dynamic, it is important to take inventory of how your work feels so that you intentionally care for yourself appropriately outside of work. These are some of the questions you can ask yourself about your workplace: Is it safe? Does the organization make any efforts to accommodate my work style? Is the setting one that places a lot of emphasis on health-related factors?

We feel more at ease and less stressed when our personal spaces are well-maintained, tidy, and organized. Being environmentally conscious improves one's health and contributes to the long-term wellbeing of society and the environment. Being able to be and feel safe is a major component of environmental wellbeing. This includes having access to clean air, food, and water; protecting the places where we live, learn, and work; living in enjoyable, stimulating environments that support our wellbeing; and encouraging study, reflection, and rest in natural settings.

Lesson: Your physical environment is often a reflection of your mental environment and that goes deeper than clutter.

For your toolbox:

Herbal medicine, also known as herbal therapy, is the practice of using plants to treat illness, improve general health and wellbeing, or to bring the body back into a state of natural balance so that it can heal itself. Different herbs have different effects on the body's various systems.

Earthing and grounding bring your body into direct physical touch with the ground. Surprisingly, lying on the ground provides health advantages that can be proven. It enables a certain electrical connection or alignment with the soil's magnetism and provides benefits comparable to antioxidants.

MOMENT OF REFLECTION
THE FEEL OF YOUR ENVIRONMENT

Task 6

When was the last time you took inventory of the feel of your daily environments?

_____

_____

_____

_____

What does it feel like when you come into your home?

_____

_____

_____

_____

How does your work environment impact your mental health?

_____

_____

_____

_____

What would give you a better sense of stability and wellness when it comes to your environment?

_____

_____

_____

_____

What is the most dominant memory regarding your adolescent environment(s)?

_____

_____

_____

_____

Do you believe you have the power to create environments that feel in alignment with your mental state?

_____

_____

_____

_____

What will you incorporate to improve your environmental health?

_____

_____

_____

_____

CHAPTER 6
PHYSICAL WELLNESS

"Good health is not something we can buy. However, it can be an extremely valuable savings account."
— Anne Wilson Schaef

To be physically healthy, one must understand the importance of getting enough exercise, eating well, and getting enough sleep, in addition to taking steps to be healthy and avoid disease and injury. Because so many of us use food as a form of self-medication, physical wellness seems to be one of the most delicate topics to broach. In our society, eating food as a form of self-medication is acceptable—unless you are obese. Yet, if you look to be in good physical shape or have a desirable body type, it is assumed that you are healthy. Let me begin by emphasizing that this is not about weight; this has to do with one's health. I recently uploaded a highlight video of my constant gym attendance over the previous year to my social media accounts. I was proud of myself because I regularly exercised. I neglected to include something significant in that post. I didn't bring up the fact that I spent a lot of money hiring a personal trainer, and after working out with him frequently for a year, I saw very little progress. You need to know that he was amazing at his job. And the lack of results was not because I didn't put in a lot of effort in the gym.

I did not see the manifestation of my work because of a sugar addiction, poor eating habits, and a lack of emphasis on my nutrition. When you put your health first, you need to do more than just go to the gym and work out. After sharing that post, I had to be brutally honest with myself. I could have kept coming up with a gazillion explanations and defenses for why I wasn't getting any results. It, however, was not going to help with the persistent exhaustion I was feeling. It wouldn't change the bloating, lack of energy, or intense sugar cravings that I was going through because emotional eating was the problem. I was using food as a form of self-medication.

When I was a young girl, my family and I would go to the store, buy all our favorite snacks, and then sit down and binge eat. I used binge eating as a release during difficult days. It developed as a conduit for challenging emotional experiences. It even served as my happy-day release. What we eat has an impact on our health. It matters what we put into our bodies. The body and mind are closely intertwined. We can think more clearly and feel more awake with the aid of a healthy, balanced diet. Moreover, it can increase and sharpen focus. On the other hand, a poor diet can cause weariness, impair judgment, and slow down reaction time. Stress and anxiety can be made worse by a bad diet and may even cause severe mental health challenges. We frequently turn to processed meals when we need a fast pick-me-up from stress or depression. Coffee replaces a full breakfast during busy or challenging times, and fresh fruits and vegetables are swapped for high-fat, high-calorie fast food. When depressed, ice cream serves as meals. I know this life-style so well because it was my life before I decided to honor my body through the foods I consume.

You are what you eat is still true, as evidenced most recently by studies into the close relationship between our intestines and brains. The vagus nerve connects our gut to our brain, allowing the two to communicate with one another physically. While the brain's emotional behavior can be influenced by the stomach, the gut's bacterial population can also be changed by the brain. One of the first stages in ensuring that your meals and snacks are well-balanced is to pay attention to how you feel after eating and what you consume. Nutritionists advise maintaining a food journal because many of us don't pay close attention to our eating behaviors.

When you sense a desire to eat, stop what you're doing, and write down your feelings if you tend to overeat under stress. You might learn what's upsetting you if you do this. Focus on consuming a lot of fruits and vegetables, as well as meals high in omega-3 fatty acids, like salmon, to improve your mental health. Vegetables with dark green leaves protect the brain. Also great for the brain are nuts, seeds, and legumes like beans and lentils. One of my favorite side effects of a well-balanced diet is the mental clarity which leads to improved decision-making. Decide to honor yourself by being more intentional about your physical health.

Lesson: Do not wait until you are sick to start prioritizing your physical health. Instead, strive towards balanced nutrition as a proactive strategy for managing your mental health.

For your Toolkit: Juicing

Our bodies require a variety of macronutrients, which we can obtain from fruits and vegetables, including calcium, minerals, zinc, and others. Our body will, therefore, receive all these nutrients if we combine different fruits and vegetables and consume them as juice. Juices contain calcium and vitamins that fortify our immune systems and shield our bodies from numerous illnesses. Juice consumption can aid in weight loss when appropriately incorporated into a diet. The quickest approach to increase your energy is via juicing. Regularly consuming fresh juice also aids to speed up your metabolism. Fruits and vegetables with leafy greens are rich in vitamin C and antioxidants. By eating a healthy diet rich in fruits and vegetables, you can reduce inflammation and remove toxins from your body. By strengthening your immune system, you can lower your risk of developing cancer. Juicing is a fast way to boost up your energy. Each fruit has its unique nutritious value.

MOMENT OF REFLECTION
HOW DO YOU HONOR YOUR TEMPLE?

Task 7

Take an honest assessment of your daily physical wellness practices. Then identify the pattern of thinking attached to your daily practices.

What are your daily exercise habits?

What is the pattern of thinking?

What are your daily eating habits?

What is the pattern of thinking?

What are your snacking habits?

What is the pattern of thinking?

What are your daily sleeping habits?

What is the pattern of thinking?

Now that you have taken inventory, what would you like to do differently?

CHAPTER 7
CREATIVE WELLNESS

"There is no doubt that creativity is the most important human resource of all. Without creativity, there would be no progress, and we would be forever repeating the same patterns."

– Edward de Bono

Though creativity is sometimes left out of lists of what wellness comprises, creating art is as crucial to wellness as eating right and exercising. I wouldn't be shocked if you were wondering why creative wellness is important. The way you express yourself artistically daily is referred to as creative wellness. I like the idea of creative wellness greatly because it used to bother me. You see, I'm the kind of person who genuinely appreciates structure. I tend to adhere to the rules more readily, and I value detailed instructions.

When I was younger, I had a distorted view of creativity. I used to believe that artists, fashionistas, and musically inclined people were the only types of people who could be considered creative. Yet, I learned that creativity is built on joy. Knowing what inspires you is important. More crucially, creative wellness is more about continuously taking care of your creative needs than it is about how you engage. Over the years, I've learned that my creativity manifests itself in the kitchen, during yoga practice, and in the way I think and believe. We may extend our viewpoints and approach difficulties from an open-minded stance when we practice creativity. Fixated thinking is the thief of creativity. Creative thought protects neurons and promotes their growth, both of which support continued cognitive function.

In his 2014 TED Talk, psychologist Mihaly Csikszentmihalyi said, "When we are engaged in creativity, we feel that we are living more fully than during the rest of our existence." This is a lovely quotation that I adore. Being creative is about expressing yourself authentically. According to the Journal of Positive Psychology, exercising our creativity enhances the performance of our immune system. It boosts good feelings while easing anxiety and depressive symptoms. When feeling stuck, our ability to enter a flow state is aided by creativity. Because of this, integrating inner child creativity into the therapeutic work with clients has been highly effective. Additionally, it enables clients to restore the younger version of themselves that was able to easily access creativity. Here are a few suggestions to help you get started:

- • Spending time in nature stimulates our emotions, which helps us think more creatively and make better decisions.
- • Painting and drawing help cope with stress and redirection, enhance memory, and build resilience.

- • Dancing and movement help to boost our mental health.
- • Singing and playing music are excellent ways to express oneself, increase oxytocin levels, and foster social connections.

Lesson: Creativity is the cornerstone for self-discovery. The act of creating something new is creative wellness. It's crucial to express your creativity since doing so may be therapeutic and can also help you understand who you are and what your passions are. You can express yourself creatively in a variety of ways, such as through poetry, dance, music, and visual art.

For Your Toolbox: Yoga

The Sanskrit word for "union" or "yoke" is yoga. To yoke is to gather, to tie, or to come together. The body, mind, soul, and global consciousness are intended to be yoked together or united in this way. Yogis can achieve profound levels of liberation, calm, and self-realization through this process of combining the physical, mental, emotional, and spiritual elements of themselves. After practicing yoga, we experience the life force flowing through our bodies, and we also feel a tangible connection to something bigger than ourselves. Original concepts and imaginative creations are born from this widened perspective.

SPEND TIME WITH CREATIVITY

Task 8.

When was the last time you planned a date with creativity? Reflect on your favorite creative activity from childhood. Did you enjoy finger painting, coloring, or cooking? Whatever you enjoyed as a child, carve out time to engage in that activity. Describe the activity below and how it made you feel when you were a child.

_____

_____

_____

_____

Describe your date with creativity?

What thoughts came up for you?

How did you show up in the creative space?

Was this time beneficial for you?

Or did you find yourself experiencing challenges with being present?

CHAPTER 8
INTELLECTUAL WELLNESS

"The concept of total wellness recognizes that our every thought, word, and behavior affects our greater health and well-being. And we, in turn, are affected not only emotionally but also physically and spiritually."

– Greg Anderson

It is simple to assume that when you hear the term, "intellectual wellbeing," it refers to education or a person's intellectual IQ, but this is not the case. The capacity to investigate and unearth new avenues for enhancing one's knowledge and abilities is referred to as intellectual wellbeing. It stems from a person's desire to study new things purely for educational purposes. Conditioning comes to mind when I think about intellectual wellness. People have been trained to learn in a very precise, constricting atmosphere, which is why this word comes to mind. We limit our intellectual experiences to taking someone else's words at face value, attending necessary professional development, or attending required academic programs. We limit ourselves when it comes to doing our own investigation or exploration.

I'm reminded of just how strong my urge to learn is when I reflect on my own experience investigating the intellectual pillar. Although I now fully embrace, accept, and adore this aspect of myself, it formerly left a large gap in my relationships. I have an endless need for knowledge. I'm one of those folks who will always be learning about life. But I found that I would frequently shrink myself in friendships and relationships because I didn't want to be the one who assumed she knew it all. A significant component of my identity and personality is intellect. I do my best in environments where I can educate and learn. I have learnt how to honor other people by not overburdening them with the things that are important or thrilling to me, even though I am no longer willing to shrink myself. To maintain my intellectual health, I look for groups of people who share my enthusiasm for learning.

A person's drive to learn through experiences like cultural events, art exhibitions, theatrical productions, and books that are outside the typical genre of literature we read is the foundation of their intellectual wellbeing. We develop our intellectual wellness when we listen and inquire about topics that are unfamiliar to us. Studying various lifestyles and keeping abreast of current events are additional strategies to doing this. Intellectual health is crucial because it enables individuals to live more balanced lives. Being knowledgeable about a range of topics helps you become more thoughtful and well-rounded. Exploration and curiosity foster intellectual wellness. Because it encourages you to try new things and gain knowledge about how you interact with others and the world around you, this curiosity is fundamental. Being aware of your connection to the environment around you helps you become a more empathic person, which improves your ability to contribute to society.

Self-discovery is critically dependent on intellectual health because conditioned creatures have a limited capacity for self-exploration. The most overused illustration of this constrained thinking, in my opinion, is when someone adopts a certain way of thinking, a practice, religion, or a belief system just because they were instructed to. Being unique beings, we have unrestricted access to information and resources. We have an obligation to fully educate and inform ourselves. Even if you educate yourself and still end up thinking in the same way that you were taught to think, you have consciously chosen that component of your identity rather than just going along with what the world thinks of you.

I've been reflecting about my path to becoming a holistic therapist. Holistic therapy was not even on my radar when I decided I wanted to be a therapist. I had a very specific perspective on therapeutic treatment. And that's how I wanted to practice therapy when I first started graduate school. It just so happened that I stumbled into a mindfulness session at my school. It was one of the least popular classes, but I was eager to learn about mindfulness. It was taught by a White woman who was very earthy and eclectic, and I remember her saying that she found it difficult to get the respect of her peers because of the method of therapy she decided to utilize. I understood what she was saying, but when I learned about the advantages of mindfulness and holistic therapy, I was really drawn to them. Years later, I work in this area as a Black woman, and I can still clearly hear what she was saying. I'm frequently taken aback by how people react to holistic therapy and by misconceptions that are founded on false information. Yet, I'm willing to share my knowledge of holistic living with others since I recognize its benefits.

Finally, intellectual wellness promotes stronger interpersonal relationships. When you make a commitment to being a student of life and view every interaction as a chance to learn more about others, people are drawn to your curiosity and your desire for friendship. Here are some tips for increasing your intellectual wellness:

- Read books purely for the purpose of education and knowledge expansion. Don't limit your reading to what is required of you; instead, read to improve your thinking and creativity.
- Immerse yourself in the musical realm. You can learn to play an instrument, learn a new musical genre, or educate yourself about a particular musical artist at any age.
- All types of games, including card games, board games, puzzles, crosswords, and word searches, improve cognitive function. Your capacity for critical thought is improved. They improve pattern recognition, which raises your social awareness.
- Go to performances that are not in your line of taste. To see what else is available, be open to trying a new type of show or concert.
- Get knowledge about different cultures' lifestyles. Discover the religious customs of others. Find out what people like to eat.

Just be curious and inquisitive because there are countless ways to live. Do not confine yourself.

Lesson: You will benefit both yourself and the world more if you continue to learn and impart your knowledge to others. You become a better version of yourself through developing your intellectual wellness.

For Your Toolbox: Hypnotherapy

Hypnotherapy is a form of therapy that uses guided hypnosis to assist a patient in achieving a trance-like state of concentration, focus, lessened peripheral awareness, and increased suggestibility. Being totally engrossed in a book, movie, song, or even one's own thoughts or meditations is what this state feels like. In it, a character exhibits remarkable receptivity to an idea or picture but is not "controlled" by anyone. Instead, a certified clinical hypnotherapist can assist clients in this condition to unwind and focus within to find and use resources that will enable them to make the needed behavioral adjustments or more effectively manage pain or other physical issues. After some time, a client learns how to handle their states of consciousness on their own, giving them more control.

MOMENT OF REFLECTION
INTELLECTUAL STIMULATION

Task 9

The goal of this task is to create an intentional plan for developing more intellectual well-being. Fill in the blanks with your plans.

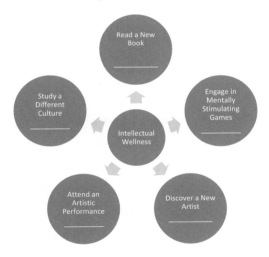

CHAPTER 9
FINANCIAL WELLNESS

"The number one problem in today's generation and economy is the lack of financial literacy."
— Alan Greenspan

Financial health, often referred to as financial well-being, is described by the U.S. Consumer Financial Protection Bureau as "the sensation of having financial security and financial flexibility of choice, in the present and when considering the future." Those who experience financial hardship can develop depression. Little symptoms may at first appear, but they can swiftly worsen, particularly if the financial situation continues to deteriorate. When past-due bills show up in the mail or bill collectors call, anxiety and sadness can spiral out of control. This may result in avoiding the issue, which would just increase anxiety and guilt. It may be quite tough to break this pattern. Stress related to money might be brought on by debt, job loss, or living over financial means.

Depending on the individual and their circumstances, each of these can lead to distinct types of depression. For instance, losing a good job can cause someone to worry about the future. These thoughts can all, to varied degrees, make you sad or anxious.

The pillar of financial wellness has really been one of the hardest for me to achieve balance in. When I was young, our primary concern was trying to survive. There was a culture of hustling to make ends meet. Hence, there were no discussions on managing credit, retiring, or even saving. Because I lacked financial literacy, very early on, I made some serious financial mistakes. Upon reflection, I can conclude that I made decisions about going to college that were fiscally immature and based on a scarcity mindset. I made the financial decision to attend a school that was much out of my league, and I asked for more student loan money than required so I may splurge and survive. I am aware that this is a widespread habit among college students, but it is fiscally immature. If I had the chance to go through that time again, I would educate myself on how to go to college without taking on debt. I would have opted for a less expensive community college that offered quality training. I would have been more prudent with the loan amounts if I needed student loans, just borrowing what was necessary to pay for my education. I'm still working on letting go of my money-related scarcity habits. The stress of inadequately managed or scarce resources can be mentally draining, which affects the wellbeing of the other pillars.

Below are the four aims of financial wellbeing. We will be closer to achieving financial wellness if we can adjust our lives to meet these financial objectives.

- Present Day Security: Establish control of your day-to-day finances.

- Future Security: Having the resources to navigate financial emergencies.

- Present Day Financial Freedom: Having the resources to financially enjoy life.

- Future Financial Freedom: Being on track to achieve long term financial goals.

Even though it is a cultural invention, money is essential to our survival. Our stress levels soar when we struggle and scrounge to pay rent, have access to transportation, and put food on the table. This isn't because we are pessimistic, emotionally unstable, or mentally ill; it's because we are wired to survive. Our tranquil times occur more frequently and last longer when our finances are in order, and we have security in the bank. Stable employment, prudent spending, and the comfort of a roof over our heads, adequate transportation, and food for our stomachs all contribute to our wellbeing.

Financial worries came in as the #1 stressor in the most recent CreditWise poll, which was released in December 2020. The research indicates that money is the leading cause of stress (73%) and is mentioned more often than politics (59%), work (49%) and family (46%). Like other types of stress, excessive financial stress can result in physical symptoms like anxiety, headaches/migraines, immune system deterioration, digestive issues, high blood pressure, muscle tension, heart arrhythmia, sadness, and a sense of being overloaded.

Here is a strategy for starting the work of improving your financial health:

- Budgeting: Your financial well-being can be built on the foundation of creating and adhering to a budget. It offers a guide for managing ongoing finances, becoming ready for monetary emergencies, and making future plans.

- Debt: Handling long-term debt and paying off consumer debt can lower obstacles to long-term financial planning, investing, and saving. The ability to responsibly manage your credit can also raise your credit score, enabling you to get better interest rates on mortgages, car loans, and other major purchases.

- Savings and Investments: For retirement planning, long-term investments and savings can offer financial security and peace of mind. Your ability to pay for anticipated expenses like holidays, house repairs, and other planned expenses with cash on hand will help you avoid taking on more debt.

- Protection and Insurance: You might be financially protected from unforeseen events by having insurance or emergency money. Losses brought on by fires, floods, or medical emergencies are all covered by insurance. Contrarily, an emergency fund provides coverage for additional situations. Both can assist in keeping you from spending your long-term savings or incurring debt.

According to Forbes, those who are under a lot of financial stress report having poor overall health twice as often and complain of ailments four times more frequently. We can improve our financial status through education, skill development, self-discipline, and wise money management. After we have achieved stability in this pillar, focusing on the other pillars of wellbeing will be easier.

Lesson: Financial wellness is achieved when we can effectively manage expenditures, pay off debt, deal with unforeseen financial emergencies, and establish plans for long-term financial goals like retirement savings.

For Your Toolkit: Breathwork

The active method of using your breath deliberately to disengage from your mind and reach another state of consciousness is called breathwork. Breathwork swiftly transports you to this state of meditation, which is what most people aim for when they sit in silence. To bypass the logical level of consciousness and enter a deeper state of consciousness, where healing, spirit, and love reside, the practice provides the brain's executive functions something to focus on. You can become conscious of ideas, feelings, memories, and patterns that aren't in line with love and self-loving while you breathe. Breathwork provides a chance to release any energy that has been unknowingly stored in the body or energetic system, even though many of us have addressed childhood, beliefs, habits, and psychopathology in therapy, coaching, or healing. There is more room for your natural life energy to circulate through you once those energies have been released.

FINANCIAL PLANNING

Task 10

The goal of this activity is to assess your current financial practices and establish a strategy for future financial wellness.

Current Practice	Future Financial Plan
Budgeting:	
Debt:	

Savings/Investments:	
Protection/Insurance:	

CHAPTER 10
SEXUAL WELLNESS

"No amount of talking about sex is going to diminish the mystery of the experience of it. Sex is Sacred, Not Secret."

— Christine Laplante, LMHC

Let's talk about sex! Well, let's discuss sexual health and wellness. The World Health Organization revised its definition of sexual health in 2006 to include "a condition of physical, emotional, mental and social well-being in regard to sexuality" rather than "just the absence of disease, dysfunction or infirmity." To put it another way, sexual health affects every facet of our lives because it lies at the crossroads of our individual psychology and biology, our family history, the health of our relationships, and a larger sociocultural framework. This means that your sexual wellbeing has less to do with the actual biological health of your individual body and more to do with the caliber of your sexual relationships, how you perceive and feel about your body and sexuality, the types of sexual behaviors you are free to engage in (including the freedom to engage in no sexual activity at all), and the types of social constraints that prevent you from leading the kind of sexual life you desire. The best way to define sexual wellbeing is a topic of discussion among academics, and wellbeing in general is difficult to define given how much it can vary within and between societies.

I had a sexual transition a few years ago. This transformation was entirely related to my sexual safety and security and had nothing to do with my sex life. It began as a desire to dress more femininely for my body type and accept my mature body. I had always carried myself modestly up until this time, so the change was significant. I had to examine how I was thinking about modesty to discover what it indicated about me. I concluded that my modesty was a reaction to sexual trauma. I experienced catcalls and sexual attempts because of my body type at a very young age. My body was the center of attention, despite the barrettes and ponytails. At age 16, I worked at a shoe store. One day when I was trying to be a model employee, a group of teenage guys walked in. We were required to put on the customary black and white shirt with black trousers, and since my shirt was tucked in, there was no way to conceal my booty while wearing that uniform. The boys requested me to help them remove a shirt from the display wall, so I had to turn my back to them to do so.

I did as they asked but felt something on my butt. I noticed the guys were giggling hysterically. When I turn around, I saw that one of the guys had placed his exposed penis on my butt after taking it out of his pants. I was startled and instantly felt ill and violated.

My coworker at the time, a male manager, made the decision to refrain from interfering. So, there were no repercussions for the sexual offense I suffered from, and the males simply departed the store. Following that, modesty gave me a sense of security. It was my coping mechanism. I always wore a large shirt or a cardigan with everything. I never felt comfortable wearing revealing clothing. And the male attention made me feel vulnerable. When I first began this transformation process, I gained knowledge from all the ways that experience transformed me, and I then reclaimed my authority by owning my sexuality. Has your sexual health changed because of any unresolved experiences?

A thorough framework for sexual wellness that spans seven domains is provided by Professors Kirstin Mitchell, Ruth Lewis, Lucia F. O'Sullivan, and Dennis Fortenberry. The results of their investigation indicated that the condition of each domain determined total sexual health. Go over the seven domains and consider how they relate to you:

- Sexual safety and security: experience with actions done to lessen vulnerability mixed with experience with threat reduction. A lack of undesired vulnerability during sexual activity, little concern about future sex life, and a sense of safety with a partner are all positive traits.
- Sexual respect: perception that one's sexual personhood is held in high regard by others. The people around you accept your sexual identity and interests, and the larger culture does as well.
- Sexual self-esteem: empathetic assessments of one's sexual self. Feeling in control of your sexual ideas and wants and positive about your physical appearance.

- Resilience in relation to sexual experiences: keeping one's balance in the face of sexual tension, dysfunctions, hardship, or trauma. Having a confidante with whom you can discuss your sexual life; needing a lot of time to recover if something negative occurs in your sexual life.

- Forgiveness of past sexual experiences: habits of self-criticism, self-shame, shame, avoidance, aggressiveness, remorse, and retaliation were stopped. Forgiveness of others and of oneself for previous sexual transgressions.

- Self-determination in one's sex life: sexual partner(s), behaviors, setting, and timing are all freely chosen or rejected without coercion, force, or a sense of responsibility. Undertaking just the sexual behaviors you truly want to express and avoiding peer pressure to engage in any sexual activity.

- Comfort with sexuality: sense of comfort in communication, introspection, and sexual expression. Focused and a sense of flow during sexual activity, the absence of undesirable thoughts, the lack of shame associated with sexual thoughts and urges, comfort with one's sexual identity and preferences, and a satisfying sexual life are all examples of these.

There are a number of things you can do to promote sexual well-being, such as communicating with your partner about your sexual needs, wishes, and desires; setting aside intentional time and space to interact sensually with your partner; looking for resources that can help you increase your sexual literacy and bust any myths you may have learned about what sex is or should be; and determining (either by yourself or with your partner) what you do and don't want from sex. In addition to everything mentioned above, it has been discovered that "sexual awareness," or the capacity to refrain from passing judgment on either yourself or your partner during a sexual experience, is one factor that is specifically linked to sexual wellbeing. Sexual mindfulness can offer sexual fulfillment, relational happiness, and self-esteem. Because sexual encounters typically produce anxiety due to the level of vulnerability required, it seems reasonable that you would have to practice being aware. It can be beneficial to practice non-judgment towards your sexual health and wellness.

Lesson: Economic stability, achieving life objectives, living longer, having better relationships, and general life happiness are just a few of the benefits that can result from having good sexual health.

For Your Toolkit: Womb Healing

The womb area can act as a holding space for unprocessed emotions. We frequently keep the energetic remnants of our traumatic experiences, emotional recollections, former partners, and relationships here. These impressions may remain hidden in our mind, which could lead to energetic barriers in the womb area. Your womb can be healed to return to its pure, unadulterated nature. The use of intuitive healing methods in conjunction with energy work, bodywork, diet, herbal remedies, and lifestyle medicine can aid in the release of emotional barriers and womb trauma as well as imprints left by prior partners. Womb healing can encourage emotional recovery from losses, including miscarriage, stillbirth, and abortions as well as assist in cutting energy cords of attachment. In womb healing, we go back to challenging memories from our past that are stored in our womb and, with the help of a knowledgeable guide, discover what beliefs were established, what emotions still need to be felt, and repair the memories to imprint new beliefs in the subconscious.

MOMENT OF REFLECTION
SEXUAL POWER

Task 11

Spend time exploring the seven domains of sexual wellness and use them to assess the state of your sexual health. Answer the questions below once you complete your assessment.

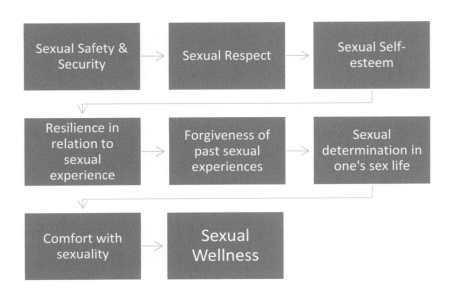

1. What did you discover about your sexual wellbeing?

73

2. What area needs more love and attention to improve your sexual health?

3. What are you willing to implement immediately?

CHAPTER 11
SPIRITUAL WELLNESS

"Getting healthy isn't just about losing weight. It's not limited to adjusting our diet and hoping for good physical results. It's about recalibrating our souls so that we want to change - spiritually, physically, and mentally. And the battle really is in all three areas."

— Lysa TerKeurst

This pillar of spiritual wellness was purposefully left till the end. The most private dimension is this one. Being spiritually healthy means having a connection to something bigger than oneself as well as a set of principles, ideals, and beliefs that give life meaning and purpose. Then allowing those principles to direct your behavior. Our ability to make decisions and judgments more easily, to remain rooted through times of change, and to develop the resilience to meet challenges with grace and inner peace are all benefits of spiritual wellness. Getting in touch with our spiritual self-aids in our recovery from both physical and emotional suffering.

I want to tell you about a time in my life when I had no spiritual grounding. I was 19 years old and had just flunked out of college. I was at the end of a long-term relationship that was becoming abusive and had no idea how to navigate life. I was suffering in silence, and I wanted it all to end. One night, I decided to act on that desire, and I consumed an enormous amount of sleeping pills. When I closed my eyes, I was confident that it would be my last day on Earth. Thankfully, my plan failed. I literally slept for hours and was angry when I woke up. When I reflect on that season of my life, I remember feeling like I was just floating and there was nothing attached to me. And because of that, I believed that my absence would not be missed.

My spiritual well-being, like most of the other pillars in my life, has been an ongoing investigation. I've given myself permission to look for meaning in varied activities and investigate many religions. I granted myself permission to go deeply into learning what speaks to me. And I've reached a place now where I feel good. My connection to my God consciousness seems very strong. My spiritual awakening provided a ton of inner peace, and I'm grateful that I finally feel as though my choices are being divinely led. I still don't have all the answers or the pieces to this puzzle; I haven't arrived. Nonetheless, I am incredibly appreciative of my knowledge of both the highs and lows, recognizing that life is just happening and that nothing is being done to make me a victim, and it's up to me to choose how I want to react. More importantly, I have a purpose, a divine assignment and I'm so grateful that I am still here to fulfill it.

For some people, spirituality means different things. As diverse as the people who pursue them are the various spiritual doctrines and practices. The variety of effects it can have on our mental health is one thing they all have in common. Our spirituality has a significant impact on our mental health. Many decisions that people make are influenced by their spirituality, and it also inspires them to develop stronger bonds with themselves. You can manage stress by turning to spirituality for a sense of serenity, purpose, and forgiveness. In times of physical or emotional stress, it frequently becomes more crucial.

Although there is no one technique to achieve spiritual wellness, all of them include leading a balanced and meaningful life. You have found peace with your life once you have reached spiritual wholeness. You view challenges as opportunities and understand that everything that happens is just a part of the journey. You can be versatile and flexible with this approach, solving issues as they appear. You can use these abilities to accomplish your goals more quickly, build wholesome relationships, make difficult choices, and be completely present to enjoy life. It is easier to attract more happiness and calm into your life when you radiate these qualities. You'll draw people to you who respect you when you have a good relationship with yourself. Leading from your heart opens the door for others to follow. The ultimate state of life mastery is spiritual wellness. Here are some ways you can work toward developing your spiritual health:

- Discover Your Purpose: Without a clear sense of purpose, you're destined to feel unfulfilled, aimless, and possibly even hopeless. Your purpose provides your life direction and significance and helps you realize that life is about "us," not "me." Serving something higher than yourself is the goal. What then is the point of living? Finding out how to enhance your spiritual wellness requires in-depth self-reflection on your needs, values, and joy-producing beliefs.

- Develop Spiritual Practices: For many of us, meditation and yoga are the first forms of spiritual wellbeing that come to mind. Make these activities a part of your daily routine if they appeal to you because they are well-liked and have been shown to be effective. You can combine aspects of meditation, visualization, and prayer. Walking outdoors, gardening, reading, keeping a journal, creating art, listening to music, and other activities are examples of spiritual practices. You can enhance your spiritual wellness by engaging in any activity that allows you to reflect and helps you feel at peace.

- Dive into Mindfulness: Being mindful is being able to pay attention to, focus on, and feel everything that is happening right now. Making thoughtful choices based on how your actions influence other people is another aspect of it. Being attentive allows you to be fully present in your life and to act morally in accordance with your values, which are two crucial elements of spiritual wellness. Start being conscious of your body, emotions, and social interactions to cultivate mindfulness.

- Spend time with Gratitude: Gratitude is a potent habit that can have a significant influence. Examining your limiting beliefs is the first step towards overcoming them. Replace these unhelpful thoughts with ones that are powerful rather than succumbing to them. Write a list of all the things for which you are thankful. Reframe unpleasant memories and consider the opportunities presented. Spiritual wellbeing is a state of mind, but it's also a set of daily acts you may practice.

- Make time for Service: One of the most effective spiritual wellness activities is giving back. It satisfies some of our most fundamental human needs, such as meaning and contribution, and it serves as a constant reminder of all the blessings we must be thankful for. Giving back helps you connect to your community and to your purpose in a way that nothing else can, whether you offer time, money, or skills. Not only will you learn the definition of spiritual health, but you'll also get to experience it for yourself.

Lesson: Wellness on a spiritual level recognizes our quest for a greater purpose in life. When our spiritual lives are in good shape, we feel more bonded to both a higher force and others around us. Our daily decisions are clearer to us, and we act in a way that is more in line with our views and values.

For Your Toolkit: Prayer and Meditation

A technique to communicate with your higher power is through prayer. By praying, you can express your faith and request assistance. Confession, thankfulness, and intercession are typically included in prayer, which is the act of communing with God (praying for the needs of others). Meditation is a type of spiritual practice that relies on concentration and limits the use of words or images. Whereas meditation does not always assume theism, prayer is understood in terms of a relationship with God. Scientific research on meditation, particularly transcendental meditation, has been extensively conducted. Transcendental meditation clearly results in a characteristic arousal pattern of relaxed alertness, and there is evidence to support its therapeutic benefits on both more objective metrics like drug and alcohol usage as well as more subjective ones like anxiety. Transcendental meditation might just be a method for deep relaxation.

MOMENT OF REFLECTION
SPIRITUAL ASSESSMENT

Task 12

Part 1. Spend some time with each of these questions to assess the state of your spiritual health.

What gives my life purpose and meaning?

_____

_____

Why am I hopeful?

_____

_____

How do I endure difficult times? Where can I find solace?

_____

_____

Am I understanding other people's perspectives on life's issues?

_____

_____

Do I try to broaden my understanding of various ethnic, racial, and religious groups?

_____

_____

Do I plan downtime into my schedule?

_____

_____

Do my decisions and behaviors reflect my values?

_____

_____

Part 2. What practices will you implement to start improving the condition of your spiritual health?

_____

_____

_____

_____

CHAPTER 12
FOCUS ON YOURSELF

"Just look at yourself in the mirror and focus on what you need to do to get better."

— Choo Freeman

Prioritizing your own needs and desires over those of other people is what it means to focus on oneself. That doesn't imply that you're intentionally trying to harm other people. It just means that you aren't sacrificing yourself to appease them. The capacity to be independent and create your own happiness is one of the most crucial talents you can master once you recognize that most people only engage on a surface level. No one will ever care nearly as much about your life as you do; therefore, you need to learn how to value your own abilities and accomplishments. When you are presented with a choice in life and thinking about what you should do, follow your heart's wishes, and pay attention to your intuition.

I hope you've figured out by now that this book is about making room in your life to perform the job of delving deeper into your existence. If you've read this far, you've probably thought about how you communicate your feelings. You've improved as a friend. You have investigated strategies to strengthen your connections with family, friends, and coworkers. I'm hoping you've decided to take better care of your physical well-being and made plans to engage in more creative activities. You have learned how to psychologically challenge yourself and get ready for financial freedom. Also, you've resolved to using your sexual power and acknowledged that you are a deeply spiritual being. Because it is difficult to look at the flawed version of self, not everyone decides to embark on this journey. Your desire to learn more about yourself, though, is admirable. Inner tranquility is the result of performing this job. I've given you a variety of tools, implement them. It is there that your world will transform.

Here are five reasons why you should focus on yourself:

- Learn your worth by putting your attention on yourself: Evaluating your self-worth is the first step in loving yourself. You are the only one who can decide it. Determine your worth, whether it be in terms of your job compensation or the durability of your relationships.

- To enhance your connections, put your attention on yourself: Others will respond with respect and honesty when you are at your most confident and are living your best life. Those who are more confident in themselves and their connections with others tend to be happier overall.

- Pay attention to yourself to identify your interests: When you put your attention on reflection, you learn which pastimes and interests bring you joy and which ones you engage in only to "fit in." You will be happy both inside and outside if you make time for the things you enjoy doing every day.

- Find your definition of success by concentrating on yourself: While the world can give you a million tips on how to be successful, everyone's idea of success is different. Be careful to give your goals a deadline when you set them for yourself. Drop it and engage in some self-discovery if it doesn't make you happy and you are doing it for someone else. Success can be defined in a variety of ways, including family, work, and travel.

- Put yourself first if you want to be happy: Positive thinking, self-worth, and confidence are the foundations of happiness. Selfishness should not be viewed as a virtue when choosing oneself over others. The entire planet would be happier if everyone was living their best lives. While everyone has a different definition of success, pleasure is a state of being that transcends all political, societal, and geographic boundaries. From the moment you get up to the moment you go to bed, put yourself first and make your own happiness your priority.

And remember, happiness and laughter are contagious. Focusing on yourself can help others focus on themselves.

ABOUT THE AUTHOR

Mrs. Tiarra Abu-Bakr is a Certified Holistic Practitioner and a Licensed Clinical Professional Counselor. A graduate of Argosy University with a Master of Art in Clinical Mental Health Counseling, Mrs. Abu-Bakr holds a Bachelor of Science in Criminal Justice from Southeastern University. True Self Holistic Therapy was founded by Tiarra Abu-Bakr. She has worked in the victim services sector for more than 15 years and is incredibly passionate about assisting people in overcoming trauma caused by issues with sexual assault, domestic abuse, infidelity, and gender identity.

In her role as a domestic violence advocate with DC Safe, Tiarra has had the chance to deal with a wide range of people for almost eight years. With the DC Department of Corrections, she devoted many years to supporting returning citizens by assisting them in reuniting with their families. As the Outreach Coordinator for the Victim Services Bureau of the Metropolitan Police Department, Tiarra had the honor of working with DC Finest to assist the families of homicide victims. Through her work, she devoted a significant amount of time to helping unhoused families and children.

Presently, Mrs. Abu-Bakr performs the duties of a mental health therapist in full, offering individual, couple, family, and group treatment. She supports people who are dealing with depression, anxiety, poor self-esteem, families going through divorce, children confronting identity issues, and girls and women who are dealing with the effects of fatherlessness. She takes a holistic approach to counseling and thinks that her clients are the ones who know best what they require; her role is to accompany them on their journey. Her areas of expertise include, women's difficulties, building healthy relationships while prioritizing sales, soul care, and juggling family, career, and self-prioritization.

Let's Stay Connected

IG: @TiarraAbubakr

Facebook: @Tiarra Abu-Bakr

Twitter: @TiarraAbubakr

Therapeutic Services: www.trueselfholistictherapy.com

Book Supplemental Resources: www.focus-on-yourself.com

REFERENCES

Adverse Childhood Experiences. (n.d.). Centers for Disease Control and Prevention. Retrieved from
https://www.cdc.gov/violenceprevention/aces/index.html

Dimensions of Wellness: Change Your Habits, Change Your Life. (2017). National Institutes of Health. Retrieved from
https://www.ncbi.nlm.nih.gov/pmc/articles/PMC5508938/

How To Tap Into The Incredible Power of Breath. (n.d.). Mindbodygreen. Retrieved from
https://www.mindbodygreen.com/articles/what-breathwork-is

Harvard Health Publishing: How to Boost Your Immune System. (n.d.). Harvard Health Publishing. Retrieved from
https://www.health.harvard.edu/staying-healthy/how-to-boost-your-immune-system

Mental Wellbeing Inherently Connected to Financial Wellness. (2021, January 22). Purdue University. Retrieved from https://www.purdue.edu/newsroom/purduetoday/re-leases/2021/Q1/mental-well-beinginherently-connected-to-financial-wellness.html

Spiritual Wellness: What is your meaning and purpose? (n.d.). Laborers' Health and Safety Fund of North America. Retrieved from https://www.lhsfna.org/spiritual-wellness-what-is-your-meaning-and-purpose/

Survey Reveals Tension in How People Think About Finances. (2021, February 2). Capital One. Retrieved from https://www.capitalone.com/about/newsroom/survey-reveals-tension-between-financial-stress-and-optimistic-financial-outlook-among-us-consumers/

The Secret to Happiness – Ted Talk. (n.d.). Ted. Retrieved from https://www.ted.com/talks/mihaly_csikszent-mihalyi_flow_the_secret_to_happiness

What is Financial Wellness? (n.d.). Annuity.org. Retrieved from https://www.annuity.org/personal-finance/financial-wellness/

What is Sexual Wellbeing and Why Does it Matter for Sexual Health? (2021). The Lancet Public Health. Retrieved from https://www.thelancet.com/journals/lanpub/article/PIIS2468-2667(21)00099-2/fulltext

Your Healthiest Self Physical Wellness Toolkit. (n.d.). National Institutes of Health. Retrieved from https://www.nih.gov/health-information/physical-wellness-toolkit

Made in the USA
Columbia, SC
01 November 2024